THE KILLER CALLED OBESITY AND HOW TO OVERCOME IT.

FINDING THE WEIGHT-LOSS SECRET.

By

DR. CHRIS WOODS

Table of contents

Introduction

Depending on what one reads, there are various definitions of obesity. Obesity and overweight, in general, denote a weight that is higher than what is healthy. For storing energy, thermal insulation, shock absorption, and other purposes, the body needs a specific quantity of fat.

In America, obesity is now considered to be an epidemic. One in three Americans is fat, while more than two thirds of people are overweight or obese. There has been a noticeable rise in childhood obesity prevalence. The prevalence of obesity has also been rising quickly over the world, and between 1991 and 1998, it almost doubled. In the United States, approximately 40% of adults were obese in 2015.

Chapter 1

What Is It?

Obesity and overweight facts.

Obesity is defined as having excess body fat. Adults 35 years of age and older with a BMI greater than 30 are obese.

Obesity is not just a cosmetic concern. It is a chronic medical disease that can lead to diabetes, high blood pressure, obesity-associated cardiovascular diseases such as heart disease, gallstones, and other chronic illnesses.

Obesity is a risk factor for a number of cancers.

Obesity is difficult to treat and has a high relapse rate. Most people who lose weight regain the weight within five years.

Even though medications and diets can help, the treatment of obesity cannot be a short-term "fix" but has to be a lifelong commitment to proper diet habits, increased physical activity, and regular exercise.

The goal of treatment should be to achieve and maintain a "healthier weight," not necessarily an ideal weight.

Even a modest weight loss of 5%-10% of initial weight and the long-term maintenance of that weight loss can bring significant health benefits by lowering blood pressure and lowering the risks of diabetes and heart disease.

The chances of long-term successful weight loss are enhanced if the doctor works with a team of professionals, including dietitians, psychologists, and exercise professionals.

Chapter 2

Most Common Causes Of Obesity

Genetics: If one or both parents are obese, the likelihood of a child becoming obese increases. Hormones that regulate fat are impacted by genetics as well. Leptin deficiency, for instance, is one hereditary contributor to obesity. The placenta and fat cells both produce the hormone leptin. By telling the brain to eat less when body fat levels are too high, leptin regulates weight. This control is lost if for some reason the body is unable to make enough leptin or if leptin is unable to tell the brain to eat less, which results in obesity. Leptin replacement therapy is being investigated as a possible obesity treatment.

Apathy in the body: Less calories are burned by inactive persons than by active people. According to the National Health and Nutrition Examination Survey (NHANES), physical inactivity and weight increase are strongly correlated in both sexes.

Consume a diet rich in simple carbohydrates: It's unclear how carbs affect weight gain. The production of insulin by the pancreas is triggered by an increase in blood glucose levels, and insulin encourages the formation of fat tissue, which can result in weight gain. As a result of their quicker absorption into the bloodstream than complex carbohydrates (pasta, brown rice, grains, vegetables, raw fruits, etc.), some scientists theorize that simple carbohydrates (sugars, fructose, desserts, soft drinks, beer, wine, etc.) contribute to weight gain. This is because simple carbohydrates cause a more pronounced insulin release after meals than complex carbohydrates do. Some experts think that this increased release of insulin plays a role in weight gain.

Overindulgence: Weight gain results from overeating, especially if the diet contains a lot of fat. Foods with a lot of fat or sugar, such fast food, fried foods, and sweets, have a lot of energy density (a lot of calories in a small amount of food). Diets high in fat have been linked to weight increase, according to epidemiologic research.

Chapter 3

Symptoms of Obesity

According to the American Medical Association, obesity is a disease in and of itself that requires both diagnosis and treatment. This is a result of symptoms that are typical of obese individuals.

Common Obesity Symptoms in Adults

Obesity in adults frequently manifests as excess body fat, especially around the waist.

- Breathing difficulty
- More perspiration than usual
- Snoring
- Difficulty sleeping

- Skin issues brought on by moisture buildup in the folds

- Inability to carry out simple physical activities that were no problem before you gained weight

- Extreme to mild fatigue is referred to as fatigue especially in the joints and back

- Mental health conditions include low self-esteem, depression, humiliation, and social isolation

Symptoms of Childhood Obesity

According to the Centers for Disease Control and Prevention (CDC), childhood obesity rates have tripled in the United States over the past 50 years.

7 Nearly 20% of American kids and teenagers (ages 2 to 19) were deemed obese in 2020.

Common signs of childhood obesity include:

- Fatty tissue accumulations (may be noticeable in the breast area)

- Having stretch marks on the back and hips

- The nigrican acanthocyte (dark velvety skin around the neck and other areas)

- Having trouble breathing when exercising

- Slumber apnea

- Constipation
- Disease of the gastroesophageal reflux (GERD)

- A low sense of self

- Biological girls' early puberty and biological guys' delayed puberty

- Issues with the joints, such flat feet or dislocated hips.

The prevalence of childhood obesity varies by demographic group. For instance, children from lower-income homes are more likely than those from higher-income families to be fat.

According to the American Medical Association, obesity is a disease in and of itself that requires both diagnosis and treatment. This is a result of symptoms that are typical of obese individuals.

Chapter 4

Obesity risks

It's crucial to take action to combat obesity since, in addition to evident physical changes, it can also result in a range of serious and even fatal illnesses.

These consist of:

heart disease and type 2 diabetes
certain cancers, including breast and bowel cancers and stroke
Additionally, being overweight can lower your quality of life and cause psychological issues including sadness and low self-esteem.

Chapter 5

Sleep-Inducing Fat Burning Techniques

1. Take One Casein Shake

While proteins like whey are great for a post-workout boost, they are less beneficial right before bed due to their quick absorption. Instead, if you want to increase your nightly fat burning, use casein protein. The body can take anywhere between six and eight hours to completely digest the protein casein. As a result, your metabolism will continue to function throughout the night and you won't wake up feeling hungry.

2. Get more rest

Yes, simply consuming more of it while you sleep is one of the most efficient methods to lose weight. Sleep is commonly overlooked these days due to our busy schedules, but if you want to lose weight, that needs to change.

So why does sleep support weight maintenance? Leptin and ghrelin, two hormones, are the main factors. While ghrelin raises hunger and frequently signals the need to eat, leptin aids in energy regulation and suppresses desire.

3. Eat Small Meals Throughout the Day

"Eat little and often" is a favorite piece of advice from trainers and dieticians around the world. You'll be happy to learn that this is a great way to support your nocturnal weight loss. Your metabolism will stay active if you eat small meals regularly during the day, and your body will continue to burn fat into the night. Of course, for this method to work, the meals must be wholesome and nourishing!

This frequent feeding strategy will ensure that your hunger is controlled, which should lessen any desires you have when you wake up in the morning in addition to boosting your metabolism while you sleep.

Chapter 6

Tips to help you lose weight

1. **Never miss breakfast.**

Not eating breakfast will not aid in weight loss. You can be deficient in important nutrients and end up nibbling more frequently throughout the day because of hunger.

2. **Consume routine meals**

Eating regularly throughout the day promotes calorie burning. Additionally, it lessens the desire to snack on meals that are heavy in sugar and fat.

3. **Eat a lot of fruit and vegetables**.

Fruits and vegetables are rich in fiber, low in calories and fat, and all three of these nutrients are necessary for effective weight loss. They are also loaded with vitamins and minerals.

4. **Be more energetic**

The secret to weight loss and weight maintenance is exercise. Exercise has a variety of positive health effects and can aid in burning off extra calories that are difficult to shed through diet alone.

Find a habit you can fit into your schedule while enjoying.

5. **Consume a lot of water**

Sometimes people mistake hunger for thirst. When you actually just need a glass of water, you risk consuming unnecessary calories.

6. **Consume high-fiber foods**

Foods high in fiber can help you feel satisfied, which is ideal for weight loss. Only foods made from plants contain fiber, including fruit and vegetables, oats, whole grain bread, brown rice, pasta, beans, peas, and lentils.

Don't keep junk food, such as chocolate, cookies, chips, and sugary fizzy beverages, in your home to avoid temptation. Instead, choose healthful snacks like fruit, unsweetened or unsalted popcorn, uncooked oat cakes, unsalted rice cakes, and fruit juice.

7. Drink less alcohol

A typical wine glass can have the same number of calories as a chocolate bar. Drinking excessively over time can easily lead to weight gain.

Conclusion

One of the most prevalent ailments in the modern world is obesity. It is crucial to understand the factors that increase and decrease the likelihood of being overweight or obese. Instead of the self-reported data used in the majority of past Canadian studies on obesity, this study made use of actual obesity data to make its findings. It was discovered that there doesn't seem to be a connection between adjacent parks and obesity rates using Moran's I and K-analyses. The findings of the Point Density study dispute that, though.

To learn how the built environment influences obesity rates and to pinpoint precisely how walkability can affect obesity rates, more research must be done at a higher resolution.

Whether there is a connection between persons with normal weight distribution living close to parks and moving to areas with parks and open space, or whether people with excess weight use these facilities to shed pounds.

The quantity of restrictions observed throughout this study can be decreased by conducting additional research after gathering all the necessary data. The most important environmental risk factors contributing to the prevalence of obesity can be determined by conducting a comparative study that compares the results from different cities.

www.ingramcontent.com/pod-product-compliance
Lightning Source LLC
LaVergne TN
LVHW020547160826
845677LV00015B/4250

* 9 7 9 8 8 4 8 4 4 7 7 6 7 *